Magic Mushroom Grower's Guide

Step by Step Guide to Learn How to Cultivate and Use Magic Mushroom

Joel Clinton

Copyright @2018

Table of contents

CHAPTER ONE

INTRODUCTION

MAGIC MUSHROOM (PSILOCYBE CUBENSIS)

The most common and easiest mushroom to cultivate is Psilocybe cubensis. This is why most mushrooms cultivators start with it. There are several methods or ways of growing mushrooms. Here, we will just consider a simple and basic method called the PF Tek Method. Pf Tek method will enable you grow magic mushrooms from scratch. This is a near perfect method that makes the cultivation of psilocybe cubensis easy, cheap and with very high success rate. This book will help you understand the dynamics of growing magic mushrooms and teach you how to prepare your PF Tek substrate and all you require to make a PF Tek substrate cakes.

Utopian Aspirations

Magic mushrooms are psychedelics which tend to generate utopian aspirations. Psychedelics tend to bring human consciousness into extreme, intense, profoundly emotional states of mystical union with all of life. This indeed can be your wake-up call. When it is taken, it's in short magical. It brings this sudden consciousness of how live on earth is and the way our society is ordered. With bourgeois propriety, hypocritical social arrangements and social conventions, you know we do live in a society that is far from been perfect which is created by men to their very best abilities. The main difference between a society and that of an animal group is that people make conscious effort to shape their society.

How does Magic mushroom grow?

The spore is an important element in which all methods begin with. A spore grows into a single mushroom, and a mushroom produces tens and hundreds of thousands of spores.

Spore prints are not only used for the identification of wild mushrooms it's also used for cultivating mushroom. Sterility is very important in all aspects of cultivating mushroom. The dry pores on the print must be hydrated before it's used. Moulds or bacteria can be used to keep them from growing together, but it can contaminate the mushroom in the process if not properly managed. Pore syringes can be purchased from suppliers if you can't make one by yourself. Relax, it is not expensive, it cost between $9 to $20 depending on the particular strain that is needed.

The following are some other equipment that are needed; canning jar, plastic container, pressure cooker or canner, vermiculite(this is a mineral gravel that is used for potting plants), brown rice flower as well as other basic kitchen items. A loose is created by mixing the brown rice flower with the vermiculite to form a fluffy substrate cake; this is a nutrient rich environment in which the mushroom pores grow. The substrate is then put in the canning jars, which are then sealed and sterilized using the canner or pressure cooker.

The jar thereafter cools after this process and the spore syringe is use to inoculate the substrate   through the holes punched in the jar's lid. The substrate is then incubated at a steady temperature of about 23.9 degrees Celsius (75 degrees Fahrenheit). In about a week the spores should begin to grow. They are called mycelium and they typically look like ropes. If nothing happens or mold grew instead then it means something went wrong.

Cakes are placed in plastic containers for fruiting, when they are covered with mycelium. The cakes in the container must have adequate light and humidity and if all goes well mushroom begins to grow after a week or two and you must be ready to pick up when the cap begins to turn upwards. Cakes normally produce muchrooms in waves and one cake can produce mushrooms for up to a month and can produce hundreds. Muchrooms can rot easily so they are either refrigerated or dried for preservation.

Cultivating mushrooms is not by any means expensive, but acquiring the spore print or syringe can be a bit difficult or challenging, this is because it is not always legal to buy.

CHAPTER TWO

12 SIMPLE STEPS TO GROW MAGIC MUSHROOMS

So many persons are scared and somehow intimidated to grow magic mushroom due to the complications involved in the process. This book will give you 12 simple steps to cultivate magic mushrooms. The method we shall be using here is the PF Tek. This is a basic grow technique that can be used to grow a wide variety of mushrooms especially the psilocybe genus.

Step1. List of Supplies Needed for Magic Mushroom Cultivation

The following are the items and requirements needed to grow magic mushroom.

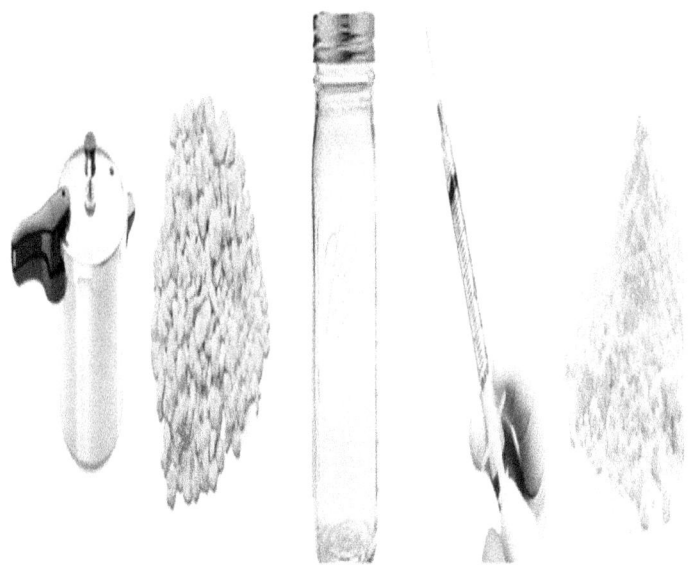

Vermiculite. Vermiculite is s medium that helps the substrate to retainin moisture. It can be gotten from big home improvement stores or small nurseries.

Pressure cooker. This is the most important equipment in cultivating mushrooms. You can browse your local thrift store to get a pressure cooker at an affordable price. The cooker is used for sterilizing your substrate so your shroom will grow to your satisfaction and produce a good yield.

Canning jars. Canning jars can be gotten from department store. half pint varieties are preferable because they are wide-mouthed with a lid.

Perlite. Perlites can be gotten from the nursery. Perlites are small white particles that maintain adequate air and improve plant respiration.

Hammer and nail. This is the easiest thing to get. Hammers and nails can be gotten from almost any shop.

Spore Syringe. This can be gotten online or from local shops. Please ensure you get a spore syringe that contain the exact strain that you wish to cultivate.

Alcohol lamp. Alcohol lamp is very important as it plays a vital role in sterilizing your needles and other materials. Please ensure it is very safe and functional.

Aquarium or large Tupperware. This serves as your humidity chamber. You can get a large sized aquarium from a thrift store for as low as $10.

Aluminum foil. If you can't get any from your kitchen cabinet, go to a nearby grocery store and get one.

Brown rice flour. Try and get the best quality of brown rice flour as this serve as your substrate from which the mycelium will feed off.

Step2. Preparing the Jars for Spore Syringes

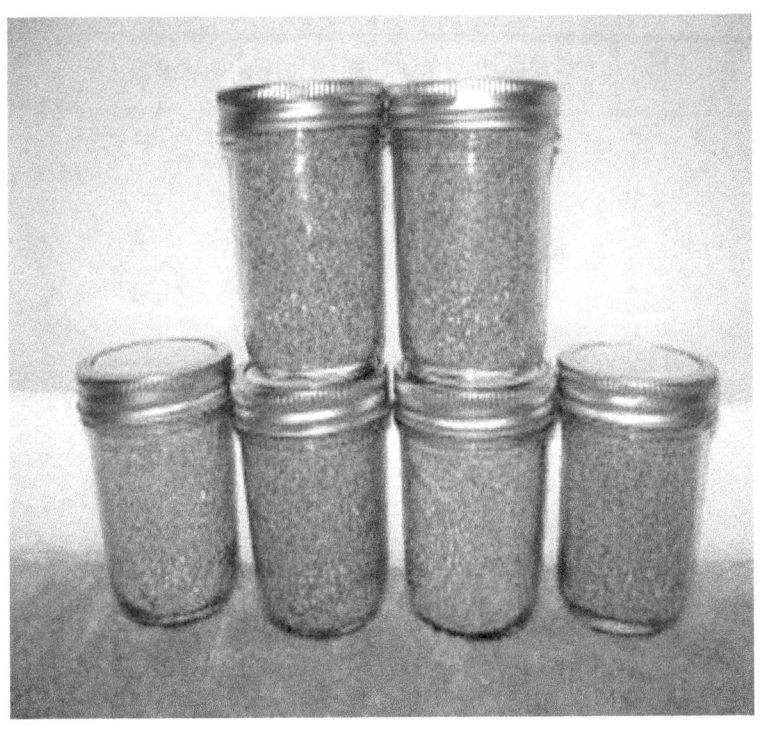

The use of spore syringes is the safest and fastest way to start your cultivation of magic mushroom. These syringes can be ordered online from various sources. Just ensure that your supplier is reliable, so you won't end up growing unwanted and undesired shroom variety.

Please ensure you use your hammer and a nail to prepare your jars by making 4 evenly spaced holes around the lid's edge. This should be done before you use your spore syringe.

Step3. Mixing Magic Mushroom Substrate

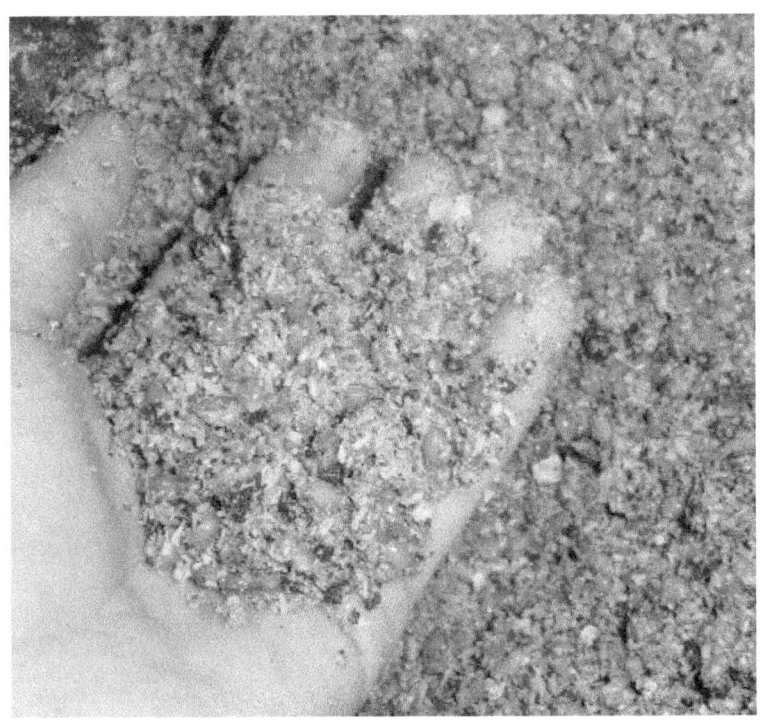

Different substances like sawdust, ground coffee, dung can be used as substrate. Since our focus here is psilocybin, we will be using brown rice flour, because they do very well with it. The substrate is what the fungus uses as its source of nutrition.

Below is a good measurement using a 8-ounce container:

- 9 cups of vermiculite
- 3 cups of substrate (brown rice flour)
- 3 cups of water

Some small amount of worm casting could also be added as it is said that worm castings do improve mushroom flushes

Step4. Filling the Jars with Substrate

Ensure you mix your moist substrate thoroughly and then pour them into the substrate jars. Then wipe off all moisture from inside and outside the jars. Please ensure you don't pack them too tightly. The jars should be loosely filled. Try and leave a space of half an inch between the top of the jar and the substrate. The remaining space should then be filled with vermiculite to provide a barrier between the substrate and the suspended microbes in the air.

Step5. Preparing the Substrate Jars for Sterilization

This step is very important. We must ensure we remove all contaminants from the jars, to avoid interference. This is like cleaning the house so that the mycelia can strive well in a good environment without unnecessary competition.

In order to prevent environmental contamination of the substrate, you have to place a square piece of foil over the lid covering the holes. To form a kind of seal over the lid, crumple the foil downward.

Place as many jars as you can inside the pressure cooker and put 3 inches of water inside the cooker. you can even stack them if you don't have enough space, but do it gently, so you don't crack the jars.

Step6. Magic Mushroom Substrate Sterilization

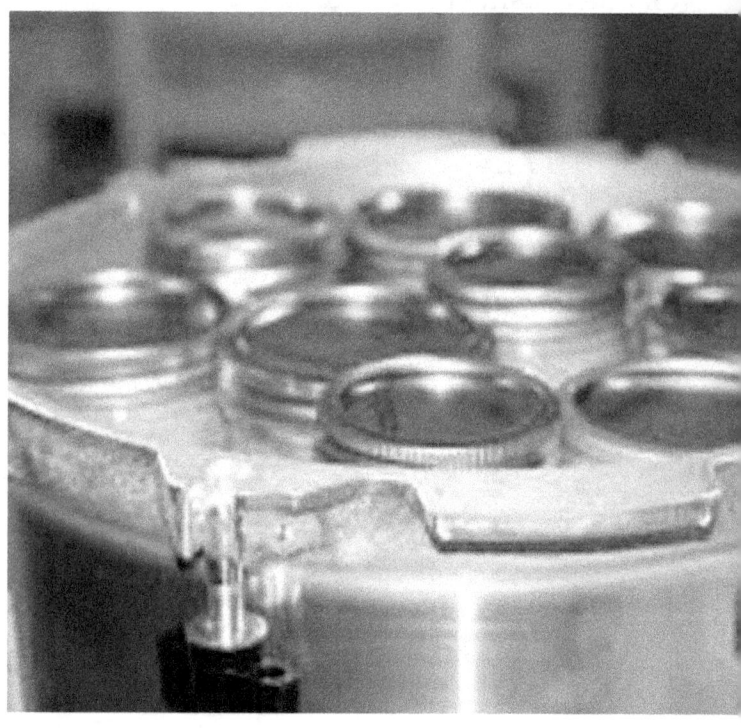

Make sure you close the pressure cooker properly, and start it up and heat when the pressure on the jars increase to 11 to 115 PSI the weight on top of the cooker or the pressure regulator starts shaking. though this depends on the manufacturer. Allow the jars to sterilize for one hour. It's preferable you do this at night so the jar can sufficiently cool before morning, and by then you will be fully ready for the next step.

Step7. Inoculating the Magic Mushroom Substrate

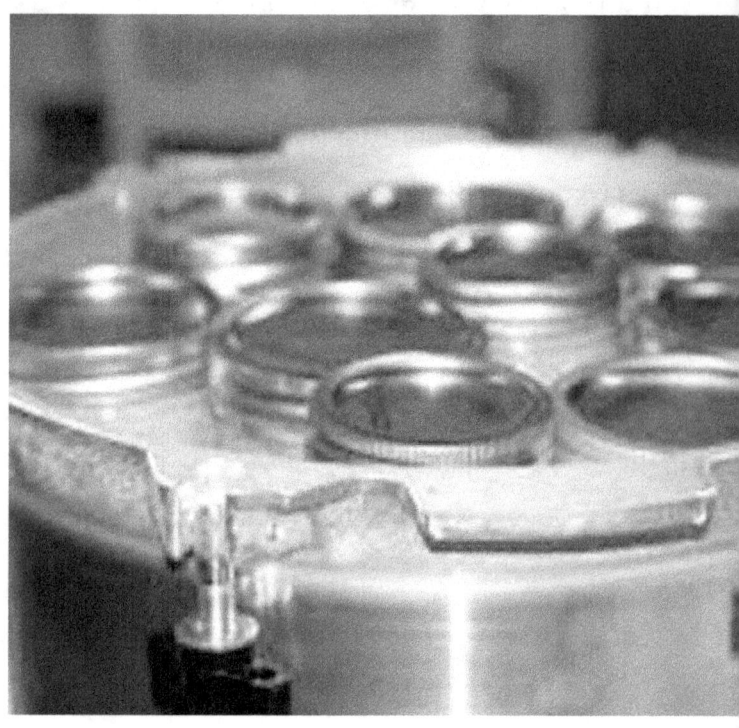

Inoculation is the process of adding spores to the sterile substrates to allow the mycelium to latch and fully develop.

You have to be extremely careful at this point, because your substrates have high tendency to be contaminated if care isn't taken. Below are the steps;

i. Remove a jar from the pressure cooker

ii. Use the alcohol lamp to heat a syringe until it becomes red hot and then let it cool for a few seconds.

iii. Remove the foil covering the hole and insert the needle of the spore syringe into the hole.

iv.   Inject approximately 1ml of the spore solution into the substrate by pushing the plunger.

v.   Repeat the process for the other jars

Here, ends the difficult part.

Step8. Incubation of the Inoculated Substrates

The mycelium is then allowed to take over the substrate and this is achieved by placing the jars in a warm and dark environment. The jars could be placed on the cupboard above your refrigerator in a cardboard box in a corner of your house. The temperature should be kept between 80 to 86 degrees F. if you can't achieve this temperature it may take little longer than necessary for mycelium to flourish. During this period mycelium will be able to absorb sufficient nutrient and water from the substrate. The first hairs of mycelium normally show up between 3 to 4days. If everything is done correctly, the fungus will colonize the substrate in 3 to 5 weeks.

Step9. Setting Up a Fruiting Chamber for the Shrooms

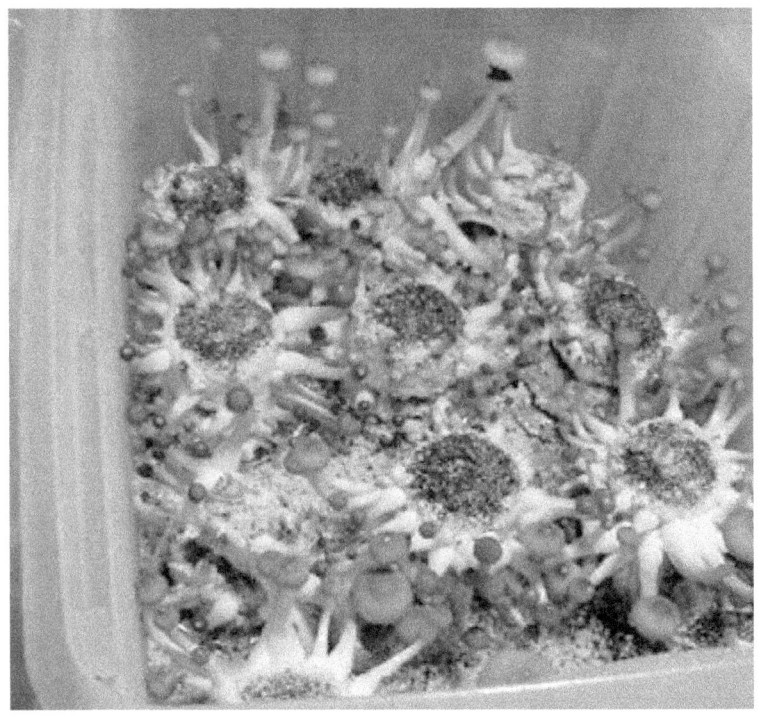

Setting up an effective fruity chamber is quite easy. The purpose is to create an environment with high humidity for the mycelium to produce fruiting bodies (magic mushrooms). You don't have to crack your head on how to get one, an old aquarium or a large Tupperware box will serve the purpose. To humidify the fruiting chamber, soak perlite in a bowl of cool water for between 5 to 10 minutes and fill the fruiting chamber with it. This set up will allow water to slowly evaporate and create an environment with high humidity inside the fruiting chamber.

Place aluminum foils on top of where you will be placing your substrate cakes. Ensure you cover the chamber very tightly. Drill some holes to allow

for air exchange. Magic mushrooms
need good amount of oxygen to
enable them survive.

Step10. Birthing the Cakes

Birthing or popping the cakes is the next step. This is a very simple process. It involves removing the lid and foil and flipping it upside down. To dislodge it, you have to give the jar a few smacks downward.

Step11. Waiting for the Flush to grow

It takes a little time for the first flush to complete growing. It may take up to two weeks depending on the mushroom strain you are cultivating.

Step12. Harvesting the Shrooms

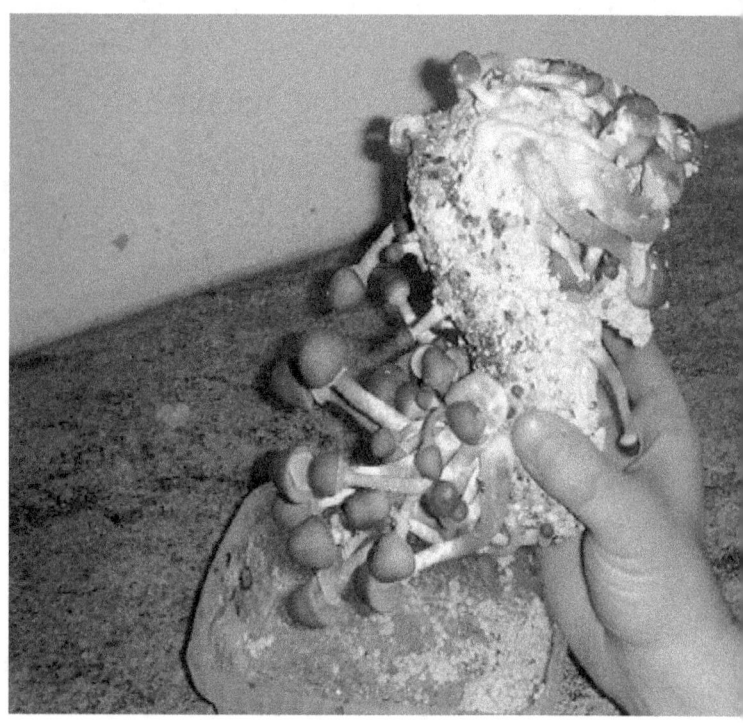

When taking your shrooms, either you cut off from the base or grab them at the base and pull.

If you follow these 12 simple steps to grow magic mushroom you are sure of having good success.

But, by peradventure if you tried and still didn't succeed, all hope is not lost. You can buy magic truffle grow kits online by using this link. magic truffle grow kits online. This kit is guaranteed to produce good psychedelic truffles in the shortest time possible with little effort.

For you to succeed in growing shrooms through either PF Tek or through a grow kit, you must be conscious of your set and setting.

Congratulations!!! You made it this far, wishing you the very best as you embark on this journey of been a big cultivator of magic mushroom and hope to hear your testimony soonest.

THE END